Anti-ageing and Skincare

Melvin Robinson

Copyright ©

Table of Contents

Reducing Wrinkles: Tips To Try First

About Sensitive Skin Care

Men's Skin Care

The Importance of Caring For Your Skin

Tips For Make Up And Skin Care

What Is Natural Skin Care?

5 Tips for Reducing Wrinkles

How to Prevent Wrinkles

Anti-Aging And Cosmetic Surgery

Cosmetic Surgery Considerations For Anti-Aging

Reducing Wrinkles: Tips To Try First

When it comes to minimizing wrinkles, you really have to consider your demands seriously. There are a lot of things that play a part in the health and well being of your skin. It is frequently hard to grasp how things function and why they may not work even though they promise to do so. If you are considering wrinkle treatments and a routine of facelifts, you may become broke in the process.

Before you accomplish all of that, consider going through a process of identifying the absolute best answer for your needs.

The first thing to consider is the health of your skin. Your skin has to be healthy if you want to protect it from looking aged too rapidly. In addition, it will assist you to seem young and healthy. Just because you have wrinkles, though, does not indicate that your skin is unhealthy. In truth, it only signifies that you need to take a deeper look at your entire health. The way to start is with your diet.

• Do you eat nutritious meals such as a diet that is rich in deep colored vegetables?
• Do you eat a lot of items that you know are not good for you?
• Do you consume meals that are extremely greasy?

All of these factors might cause various regions of your body to not work in the appropriate way. If you are seeking a remedy to your wrinkles , start with adjusting your overall diet. This implies giving your body the appropriate nutrients through the food that you consume. Many people make the mistake of believing that what they eat doesn't matter. If you are obtaining wrinkles early on, it might be caused by your lack of a balanced diet. Enhance your nutrition and improve your general health as well as your skin's appearance.

Reducing Wrinkles: Improving Your Skin's Look

When it comes to eliminating wrinkles, one of the first things that you should do is identify how you can enhance all of your skin on your face and neck area. Although some wrinkles are linked to age, the condition of your skin is an essential issue, too. In many aspects, it is vital to take the time to repair the problems with your skin if you want to change the way that wrinkles impact your appearance. In fact, healthy skin will be beneficial in the long run with less wrinkles if you enhance its health today.

One thing that you should do to achieve this is to provide your skin the correct nutrients. Now, most of the diets that Americans consume are not the finest in quality and tragically, even when they are thought out and carefully planned, they still do not carry enough of a punch to enhance our health. In many circumstances, it will be required to consider adding more nutrients to your diet to discover actual improvement.

You will want to throw in an excellent multivitamin. Visit your local health foods store, or better yet discover a trusted provider online. Purchase a very excellent grade multivitamin. Those that are oriented on providing for older individuals are not always going to be better for you. Whatever you do, try putting in a decent concentration of Vitamin A, Vitamin C, and Vitamin E.

These are top grade antioxidants. In your bloodstream, things called free radicals exist. These may be thought of as little particles that you breathe in. They not only can pile up and develop life threatening illnesses, but they also block your cells and cause your skin to seem unhealthy.

To lessen the wrinkles on your skin, increase the health of your skin by providing it the nutrients that it requires to have to survive. The good news is that this process doesn't have to be tough at all.

Reducing Wrinkles Through Exfoliating

You have heard about the chemical peel and it sounds much more terrible than it is. But, what if you could obtain the advantages of the chemical peel at home and lessen the wrinkles that are on your skin? There are innumerable ways that this may help you, in fact. If you are not included in a regular routine of natural and soothing cleansers, do that first. Then, consider throwing in an exfoliating product, too. When you do this, you increase the general quality of your skin, giving you a very excellent appearing attractiveness.

Foremost things first, examine your cleansing approach. You should be putting a solution on your face each day and night. What you don't want to do is to use hand soaps or soap bars to wash your face. These creams remove much too much of the extremely crucial natural oils on your skin, leaving it dry and even cracked. This skin is not healthy, it aches and it is more likely to lead to more problems with wrinkles in the future. Purchase a good grade cleansing routine that is friendly to your skin.

Then, exfoliate. This is a method that merely removes the very top layer of skin on your face quickly, lightly and actually without discomfort. It also helps to eliminate the dead skin cells there, as well. When it accomplishes this, it will safely prompt your skin to do something about the need to replace this skin. When fresh skin grows back in lieu of what you removed, it is younger and much more healthy. In fact, it is less wrinkled, too.

When it comes to increasing the condition of your skin, regular bathing is crucial. Make now the opportunity to indulge a little on you. Invest in a quality product that is capable of supplying you with the aid you need. Exfoliating is also a major element. Do these activities and improve wrinkles.

Reducing Wrinkles: Stay Out Of The Sun

Before you run off to purchase a highly costly wrinkle cream, take a look at the manner that you are managing your skin. No matter what the cream is that you plan to use, if you do not take care of your skin in the first place, it can't work for you. Many individuals make the error with utilizing a wrinkle cream as a band aid, but that band aid might not function if you don't tackle the cause first. But, before you can accomplish that, you have to analyze your existing circumstances.

Many people develop wrinkles because of the sun. The sun's rays are destructive to our bodies. For most of us, the concept of applying sun protection only comes into play on those days when the beach is the goal or when the summer weather is in full force. The trouble is that even on gloomy days or in the dead of winter, the UV rays are reaching through and hurting your skin. The more exposure that you have, the more likely you are to need to do anything to remedy it. Not only is UV radiation the biggest cause of skin malignancies, but it is also a factor behind the wrinkle, too.

So, what do you do? Look for make up items that feature UV protection. Or, apply sunscreen to your skin before applying anything else. Make sure that when you head out of the house each day, you do the same for your children. The reality is that your skin requires sunscreen if you wish to appear your age or younger. If you don't use it or don't apply it often enough, you run the danger of confronting sun damage and wrinkles are part of that bundle. Don't allow your skin to suffer from these problems. Help stop the wrinkles from appearing using sun protection.

Reducing Wrinkles: Choices To Consider

Once you have taken the time to enhance your body's general health and well being, the next stage in the process is increasing the quality of your skin through various ways. There are various solutions out there that can substantially or marginally aid you to enhance your skin and lessen your wrinkles. Each of these approaches has worked for some but there is no assurance that any regimen will work for you. Talking with your dermatologist and your cosmetic surgeon is the best method to evaluate your possible benefit.

Here are some alternatives.

• Wrinkle creams. These are widely available and can work for you. To make sure you receive one that is useful, check for ones that include Retinal. They should state this or they should indicate they include Vitamin A, Vitamin C, and Vitamin E. Products that profess to be miracle products are not likely to be very useful, though.

• Botox. This is one of the heavily promoted products nowadays for reducing wrinkles from the face. If you are interested in finding a remedy that is least intrusive, this is the ideal one. But, remember that you may need to get it updated regularly. It is an easy decision and one that can be done during your lunch hour.

• Face lift. The face lift is a considerably more extreme choice, but it doesn't have to be. There are many smaller sorts of modifications that may be done to aid increase the skin's capacity to appear wonderful. Small and significant modifications might be done to erase the wrinkles in your skin.

These are just some of the numerous sorts of treatments that are available to you to enable you to enhance your skin. Take the time that it takes to find the ideal one that meets your requirements and the budget that you have.

About Sensitive Skin Care

'Sensitive skin care' is controlled by a few simple criteria. However, even before we dig into the principles for sensitive skin care, it's necessary to grasp what a sensitive skin is. Sensitive skin is one which is unable to endure any unfavorable conditions (environmental/other), and which readily becomes irritated on contact with foreign materials (including skin care products) (including skin care products).

For this reason, several products are particularly branded as sensitive skin care products. The degree of sensitivity might nevertheless vary from person to person (and based on that, the sensitive skin care techniques vary too) (and depending on that, the sensitive skin care procedures vary too).

Generally, all skin types respond unfavorably to detergents and other chemical based products. However, the harm starts typically above a set threshold (or tolerance level) (or tolerance level). This tolerance level is quite low for sensitive skin types, leading to skin becoming harmed very easily and fast. Sensitive skin care products either avoid the possible irritants or keep them at extremely low doses.

Here are a few recommendations for sensitive skin care:

* Use sensitive skin care products only (i.e. the items that are indicated for sensitive skin care only) (i.e. the products that are marked for sensitive skin care only). Also, examine the instructions/ notes on the goods to determine if there are special restrictions/warnings linked with the product).

* Even within the spectrum of sensitive skin care products, pick the one that contains fewest preservatives, colorings and other chemicals
* Do not use toners. Most of them are alcohol based and are not suggested for delicate skin.
* Wear protective gloves when doing laundry or other chemical based cleaning. If you are allergic to rubber, you can wear cotton gloves below the rubber ones.
* Another key suggestion for 'sensitive skin care' is to prevent excessive exposure to sun. Apply sunscreen cream before heading out in the sun.
* Avoiding exposure to dust and other contaminants is also vital for sensitive skin care. So, cover yourself fully before heading out.
* Use hypoallergenic, non comedogenic moisturizer as a sensitive skin care product (if there is none particularly labeled as a sensitive skin care product) (if there is none

specifically labeled as a sensitive skin care product)

* Use soap-free and alcohol free cleaners. Cleanse your face anytime you return from spending time out doors.\s* Do not scrape or exfoliate too hard. It can produce reddishness and possibly inflammation.\s* Do not keep the makeup on for too long. Use hypoallergenic makeup- removers.

So, sensitive skin care is extremely different from the typical skin care. Sensitive skin care is more about being careful with your skin (both in terms of sensitive skin care products and protection against surroundings brutality on skin) (both in terms of sensitive skin care products and protection against environmental atrocities on skin).

Anti-Ageing Skin Care

'Anti-ageing skin care' is a highly common notion in today's globe. Today everyone wants to mask their age with anti-ageing skin care techniques (and a lot of individuals are successful too) (and a number of people are successful too). However anti-ageing skin care is not achieved by any miracle remedy. 'Antiaging skin care' is about discipline. It is about being proactive. Antiaging skin care is retarding the ageing process. Here are a few recommendations for proactive anti-ageing skin care:

1. Maintain healthy eating habits: A properly balanced diet is the key to maintaining a normal body metabolism. Eat a lot of fruits and vegetables (raw), they are the best source of fibre and have a highly refreshing impact on your body. Avoid greasy and fatty meals; not only do they lack in important nutrients but also induce obesity and other ailments which help the aging process

2. Beat stress: This is perhaps the most significant anti-ageing skin care measure. Stress disrupts the biological metabolism and increases the aging process. Sleep, exercise and a soothing bath, are all wonderful techniques of overcoming stress. Aroma-therapy is also proven to bust tension.

3. Drink a lot of water: Antiaging skin care can't be much easier than this. Water aids in draining out the toxins from the body, thereby keeping it clean and making it less prone to disease. Around 8 glasses of water (per day) is suggested by all doctors.

4. Regular exercise is a superb anti-ageing skin care technique. Besides toning your muscles, it also assists in cleansing the skin by draining out the toxins in the form of perspiration. Exercise should be followed by a warm shower in order to totally eliminate the toxins.

5. Avoid the use of harsh, chemical based products on your skin. Natural skin care products are a fantastic alternative. Use of organic skin care products (home produced or commercial) can be a very effective anti-ageing skin care strategy.

6. Do not overdo skin care products. Excessive and severe application, both are dangerous.

7. Do not neglect skin issues; it can lead to irreversible skin damage. Try over the counter medicine and if it doesn't help, immediately contact your dermatologist and ask his/her advise.

8. Vitamin C based skin care products are particularly popular ways of anti-ageing skin care. However, they tend to oxidize quite fast (which makes them toxic for the skin)

(which makes them harmful for the skin). So keep them correctly. If the product turns Yellowish brown, it implies that vitamin c has oxidized and the product is no longer appropriate for usage.

9. Protect your skin against UV radiation; UV rays are believed to speed up the aging process. So, an excellent sunscreen lotion should be a component of your anti-ageing skin care regimen.

Herbal Skin Care

Skin care is not a topic of modern times; it has been in use since ancient times, when herbal skin care was perhaps the only means to take care of skin. However, skin care has altered in a dramatic manner. Herbal skin care procedures have been supplanted by synthetic/chemical-based skin care routines. The herbal skin care recipes which formerly used to be commonplace are not so popular anymore (and even unknown to a huge public) (and even unknown to a large population).

This change from herbal skin care to synthetic, may probably be ascribed to two factors - our laziness (or just the quick pace of life) and the commercialization of skin care. Even natural skin care products have been marketed. These commercial herbal skin care products have to be blended with preservatives in order to improve their shelf-life, thereby making them less effective than the fresh ones created at home.

However, it seems that things are changing fast and more people are now opting for natural and herbal skin care routines. But still, none desire to produce them at home and why the commercial industry of herbal skin care products is on the increase.

So what are these herbs or natural skin care mechanisms?

Aloe Vera, which is an extract from the Aloe plant, is one of the greatest examples of herbal skin care product. Freshly harvested aloe Vera is a natural hydrant that aids in healing skin. It also aids in mending injuries and repairing sun burns.

A variety of plants are recognized to contain cleaning qualities. Dandelion, chamomile, lime blossoms and rosemary herbs, are a few examples of such cleansers. Their herbal skin care qualities become activated when they are coupled with other herbs like tea.

Antiseptics are another key aspect of Herbal skin care. Lavender, marigold, thyme and fennel are wonderful examples of plants that are known to contain antibacterial characteristics. Lavender water and rose water also create effective toners.

Tea plays a vital position in herbal skin care. Tea extracts are utilized for therapy of skin that has been affected by UV radiation.

Oils derived from herbal extracts give additional approach of natural skin care. Tea tree oil, Lavender oil, borage oil and primrose oil are some prominent oils used in herbal skin care. Some

fruit oils (e.g. extracts from fruits like banana, apple and melon) find application in shower gels (as a moisturizing combination) (as a hydrating mix)

Homeopathic treatments and aromatherapies also come under the banner of herbal skin care solutions.

Herbal skin care is beneficial not only for the usual nourishment of skin but also for treatment of skin problems like eczema and psoriasis. Most herbal skin care products don't have any adverse effects (the most essential argument for preferring them over synthetic treatments) (the most important reason for preferring them over synthetic products).

Moreover, herbal skin care products may be simply created at home, thereby making them even more attractive. So, natural skin care is the way to go. However, this does not mean that you fully disregard the synthetic items. Some people go to the level of disagreeing with their dermatologist, if he/she advises a synthetic product. You should acknowledge the reality that some skin types can necessitate utilization of clinically proven non-herbal skin care products.

Men's Skin Care

"Man skin care" may appear like an exotic issue to some males. It would have been much more strange a few years back. However, more and more guys are increasingly discovering the necessity of men's skin care (which is why you find marketplaces flooded with male skin care products too) (and hence you see markets flush with man skin care products too). Even though the male skin is substantially different from that of a female, "man skin care" is fairly comparable to skin care for women.

"Man skin care" too starts with washing. Water-soluble cleaners are preferable. Cleaning helps eliminate dirt, oil, and impurities from the skin and assists in avoiding pore blockage. The natural oily condition of male skin makes cleaning a crucial aspect of a man's skin care routine.

Cleansing should be done at least once per day, even better if it is done twice a day. Using soap on the face is discouraged.

"Man skin care" revolves a lot around shaving. Shaving foam/gel/cream and after shave lotion are two of the most significant male skin care items. Serious Man skin care' demands a suitable selection of shaving-related equipment and supplies. One of the primary factors in choosing shaving products should be skin type (because the degree of oiliness changes from person to person), since the degree of oiliness differs from person to person. Alcohol-based aftershaves should be avoided.

Proper "man skin care" also necessitates the use of top-grade razors. Here, swivel-head razors are favoured as they are known to reduce cuts. Besides these items and equipment, it is also vital that you use them appropriately. Be gentle when using your razor. Do not scratch it against your skin; use a light and smooth movement (after all, it's a question of eliminating hair, not the skin itself).

Male skin is often thicker and oilier, owing to wider pores and more active sebaceous glands. However, owing to continuous shaving, the skin can get dry rather readily. Hence, moisturizers to form a vital aspect of men's skin care. Moisturizing gel or cream should be administered after shaving. In reality, certain shaving foams or gels have an in-built moisturizing function too. Moisturizers should be rubbed softly over the face and massaged gently upwards.

Though a guy's skin is less vulnerable to skin cancer caused by UV radiation, employing a sunscreen is nonetheless a vital male skin care practice. You can use a moisturizer that combines sunscreen with a hydrating effect.

Another fantastic choice for "men's skin care" is to utilize male skin care products that include natural components like aloe vera, sea salt, and coconut oil. Naturally antibacterial oils, e.g. lavender, tea tree, etc., also give ideal methods for male skin care.

Mankind's skin care is not as tough as a lot of men assume. It merely takes just a few minutes every day in order to provide you with healthy skin for today and for the future.

"Personal Skin Care" Is A Routine

We all know the importance of "personal skin care." The opinion on how-to (for personal skin care) changes from person to person. Some individuals assume that attending beauty parlors every other day is personal skin care. Others feel that personal skin care is only a question of applying some cream or lotion to your skin every now and then.

Then there are those who assume that personal skin care is an event that happens once a month or once a year. Still others concern themselves with "personal skin care" all the time. However, personal skin care is not that hard and neither is it that expensive (given how good it is) or how beneficial it is. Personal skin care is following a regimen or a method for caring for the needs of your skin.

Even before you start with a routine, you need to assess your skin type (oily, dry, sensitive, normal, etc.) and pick the personal skin care products fit for it (you might have to trial with a few personal skin care products) (you might have to experiment with a few personal skin care products). Here is a regimen that should work for most people with regular skin.

The first item in your personal skin care routine is "cleansing." The three primary constituents of a cleaner are oil, water and surfactants (wetting agents). Oil and surfactants take dirt and oil from your skin, and water then washes it out, thereby making your skin clean. You might have to test a number of different cleansers before you locate the one that suits you the best. However, you should always use soap-free cleaners. Also, you should use lukewarm water for cleansing (hot and cold water do damage to your skin) (hot and cold water both cause damage to your skin). Take care that you don't over-cleanse your skin and wind up hurting it in the process.

The second thing in the personal skin care routine is exfoliation. Skin has a natural maintenance process wherein it eliminates dead cells and replaces them with new skin cells. Exfoliation is only a means to aid the skin in this process. Dead skin cells are not capable of reacting to personal skin care products but still eat these items, thereby preventing them from reaching the new skin cells.

Thus, eliminating dead skin cells is crucial in order to boost the efficiency of all personal skin care products. Generally, exfoliation takes place shortly after cleaning. As with any personal skin care technique, it's crucial that you understand how much exfoliation you require. Exfoliate 4-5 times per week for oily or normal skin and 1-2 times per week for dry or sensitive skin. Exfoliate a couple of times more in hot and humid conditions.

The next thing in your personal skin care routine is moisturizers. This is one of the most crucial aspects of personal skin care. Even those with greasy skin require moisturizers. Moisturizers not only seal the moisture in your skin cells but also draw moisture (from air) whenever needed. Use of too much moisturizer might clog skin pores and end up hurting your skin. The amount of moisturizer needed by your skin will become evident to you within one week of you utilizing the moisturizer. Also, applying the moisturizer is ideal when your skin is still damp.

The final thing in your personal skin care routine is sunscreen. A number of moisturizers (day-time creams or moisturizers) come with UV protection, so you can receive double advantages from them. Such moisturizers are advised for all days (irrespective of whether it is sunny or gloomy) (irrespective of whether it is sunny or cloudy).

Again, try with various personal skin care products and also with the amount you need to use. What provides you with the greatest results is the finest personal skin care formula for you. However, if you have any type of skin difficulty, it is important to see your dermatologist before you really start utilizing any personal skin care products.

Serious Skin Care

"Serious skin care" is about preserving healthy and bright skin all your life. As you get older, your body's natural skin care functions become weaker. So, "serious skin care" is about adapting to the changing demands of your skin. Thus, "serious skin care" is about regularly reviewing, analyzing, and adjusting your skin care procedures. Your skin care routine should fluctuate depending on the ambient circumstances, your age, and changes in your skin type.

"Serious skin care" is also about awareness. With technological breakthroughs and studies, more and more facts are being brought to light every day. Also, the content and type of skin care products seem to be evolving with time. So checking out the new products is also a component of serious skin care. However, "serious skin care" suggests using a new product on a tiny patch of skin (not your face skin) first, merely to observe how your skin reacts to it.

"Serious skin care" also entails learning how to utilize your skin care products. Good practices include things like applying the moisturizers when the skin is damp, using upward strokes for greater penetration of skin care products, removing the make-up before going to bed, washing before moisturizing or putting on make-up, using the proper amount of skin care products, etc. Thus, enhancing the effectiveness of your skin care products is another focal area of serious skin care.

Some measures, such as avoiding contact with detergents, are also part of serious skin care. "Serious skin care" implies being careful with your skin. Things like over-exfoliation, usage of low quality products, and application of strong-chemical-based treatments are all detrimental to your skin. Some individuals have a mistaken notion about serious skin care. For them, serious skin care means using enormous quantities of cosmetics as often as possible. However, this truly isn't serious skin care (and that's why awareness is so crucial).

"Serious skin care" is also about consulting your dermatologist for treatment of skin diseases. Ignoring skin diseases may be disastrous for your skin and could lead to irreversible damage. So, if the items don't improve with over-the-counter medicine, you should promptly consult a dermatologist. Self-surgery, such as squeezing acne/pimples, is a big no (it can cause irreversible damage to your skin) (it can cause permanent damage to your skin).

So, very serious skin care is more about precautions and preventive measures (than therapy) than treatment. Serious skin care is about being preventative as well as reactive. In fact, we may say that "serious skin care" is about being proactive about the requirements of your skin so that the necessity for being reactive is kept to a minimum.

Skin Care Cosmetics—Useful Or Harmful?

A beautiful and healthy skin is a major confidence booster. Some individuals are inherently gorgeous and consequently don't use any "skin care cosmetics." Then there are those who don't apply skin care cosmetics owing to their laziness. Still, some feel that skin care cosmetics might hurt their skin, and so forsake the usage of any form of skin care cosmetic. However, there are a huge number of individuals who do utilize skin care cosmetics (that's why the industry of skin care cosmetics is thriving).

So, is skin care cosmetic helpful or harmful?Well, the opinions appear divided. However, one thing is for sure: looking gorgeous is undoubtedly great and quite desirable. Furthermore, an excess of skin care products is undoubtedly hazardous (as such, an excess of anything is toxic) (as such, an excess of anything is harmful).So, what does one do?

The first step is to develop (and maintain) a skin care program that will help keep your skin healthy and disease-free. The usual guideline is to wash and moisturize regularly, then tone and exfoliate occasionally (as and when needed).

The next item is the skin care cosmetics that you would be utilizing additionally (as beauty boosters) (as beauty enhancers). These skin care cosmetics might either be part of your skin care regimen or be applied exclusively for special occasions (e.g. while attending a party etc).

The most crucial thing about skin care cosmetics is their choice. Here is a list of principles that you should apply while picking any skin-care cosmetic:

The basic rule is to use cosmetics that match your skin type. This is true both for the regular goods and for the skin-care cosmetics. So check the label to see what it says, e.g., 'for dry skin only' or 'for all skin types' etc.
* Test the skin care cosmetic before using it. This may be done by applying the skin care product to a small patch of skin, e.g., ear lobes, and observing the reaction of your skin to the product. * Check the components of the skin care product for chemicals that you are allergic to. Do not use items that are extremely harsh on the skin, such as products with high alcohol concentrations;

such cosmetics may work temporarily but cause long-term harm to your skin.

* 'More isn't better'. Make sure you use the correct amount of each item (neither less nor more).Also, be careful with your skin and follow the appropriate techniques for application of skin care products. Rubbing too hard or trying to squeeze a pimple might lead to irreversible harm to your skin.ss * Finally, if you have a skin disorder, e.g., acne, you should consult your dermatologist before using any skin care product.

The Importance of Caring For Your Skin

"Packaging is as essential as the present itself"—it's something that most of the gift production firms observe very seriously. The same holds true for you too. Your outer-self, i.e., your skin, is as vital as your inner-self. A lot of individuals do recognize the importance of skin care. Well, this is one reason why there are so many skin care products on the market and most of them seem to do very well. We often prefer to link skin care to merely excellent appearance. However, there is more to it than simply that. There are various benefits linked with having healthy and bright skin.

Firstly, it has a favorable influence on you personally. It helps you feel fresh and active. You are able to complete more work and are speedier with all you do. More significantly, the freshness adds to your delight and enhances your day. So a healthy skin too plays its part in generating confidence. Yes, you may claim most of the credit for having done that (although do leave a bit for the skin care products too) (however, do leave a little for the skin care products too).

Moreover, this flow of pleasant energy is felt by individuals around you also, and you realize that they are nicer to you. You will acquire greater respect from others. They are more receptive to your inquiries. They themselves sense the freshness that you are emitting.

They adore working with you and for you. Yes, that's how it works. Some folks could even go ahead and question you about the skin care products you use (you might or might not share those secret skin care products with them) (you might or might not reveal those secret skin care products to them). Thus, having a healthy skin may be important in generating a pleasant and welcoming atmosphere around you. On the other hand, carelessness or negligence on this front might make you seem unappealing and uninterested. You will not only appear drab but also feel dull. Your job efficiency is diminished. Even the individuals you encounter might not be as nice. In fact, it may contribute to the aging process starting much sooner.

Thus, the necessity of skin care cannot be overlooked. However, skin care is not that tough at all. There are a lot of skin care products available, and you may select the ones that fit you the best. There are different methods in which skin care products are categorized, and the information about these categories will help you understand them better and make a choice.

* The first category is based on skin type; thus, you have oily skin care products, dry skin care products, sensitive skin care products, and so on.

* Another option is to categorize skin care products based on their intended use, such as moisturizers, cleansers, exfoliation products, toners, and so on.

* Then you have skin care goods for therapy of various skin issues i.e. skin care products for acne, skin care products for stretch marks, skin care products for anti-ageing etc.

* Another classification is based on the ingredients, e.g., herbal skin care products, synthetic skin care products, cosmetic skin care products etc.

However, skin care products are not the sole means of skin care. You also need to develop some basic skin care practices in your day-to-day life (as we cover in the other post on personal skin care) (as we discuss in the other article on personal skin care).

Skin Care Treatment For The Most Common Skin Conditions

A beautiful and healthy skin is an advantage. Skin is not all about appearance but also health. So, skin care therapy should be addressed with utmost attention. If you acquire a skin related difficulty, you require a suitable skin care therapy. Skin care therapy, for any skin problem, starts with measures that are intended at prevention of the disorder (what we may also term as proactive or preventive skin care treatment) (what we can also call as proactive or preventive skin care treatment).

Building and implementing fundamental skin care practices is what one may categorize as preventive/proactive skin care treatment. Skin diseases might emerge even if you have followed this preventative skin care regimen. Preventive skin care therapy only minimizes the risk of occurrence. Let's explore the skin care therapy for some of the prevalent skin disorders.

Acne is one of the most frequent problems. Again, the primary form of skin care therapy is to manage acne and prevent it from growing worse. So avoid tight garments; they are known to induce body acne by trapping perspiration. Do not touch the imperfections over and over again (better don't touch them at all), you can wind up exacerbating the disease. Also, do not try to scrape too hard or pressure them. Use of gentle cleansers is a suggested skin care therapy for acne. Obtain an over-the-counter skin care medication for speedier treatment of acne.

Skin care treatment of dry skin is often uncomplicated. Moisturizers, applied in the proper technique and in the appropriate quantity, are the greatest kind of skin care treatment for dry skin. For optimal results, use moisturizer when your skin is still wet. Also, do not use too much or too little moisturizer. In rare circumstances, when you don't observe any changes in 3-4 weeks, you might have to contact your dermatologist for skin care treatment of your dry skin.

Brown spots, which occur on sun-exposed parts of skin i.e. face and hands, are produced by over-exposure to UV radiations. As a skin care therapy for brown spots, apply a sunscreen lotion which has a high SPF (sun protection factor), say 15. This should be used irrespective of weather - sunny/cloudy. Another kind of skin care therapy is covering up the exposed portions with clothes (caps, full sleeved shirts/t-shirts, and umbrella).

Also, if the general skin care therapy or the over-the-counter medicine is not working for you, you should immediately contact your dermatologist for expert skin care treatment. You should also notify the doctor about the skin care therapy that you have performed till

that time. So carry the information of the till-date skin care therapy (and products) along with you. Based on the skin condition and the specifics of your till-date skin care therapy, the dermatologist will recommend a skin care treatment e.g. oral antibiotics, chemical peels, retinoid etc and you will be on your path to recovery.

The Facts About Oily Skin Care

To start the conversation on oily skin care, it's necessary to first grasp the cause behind oily skin. Put simply, oily skin is a result of excessive production of sebum (an oily material that is naturally generated by skin) (an oily substance that is naturally produced by skin). As is known to everyone, excess of anything is bad; therefore excessive sebum is harmful also. It leads to blocking of skin pores, leading in accumulation of dead cells and consequently production of pimples/acne. Moreover, greasy skin ruins your appearance too. So, 'oily skin care' is as necessary as the 'skin care' for other types of skin.

The main purpose of 'oily skin care' is the elimination of excessive sebum or oil from the skin. However, oily skin care techniques should not lead to full elimination of oil. 'Oily skin care' starts with the use of a cleanser. However, not all cleaners will work. You need a cleanser which contains salicylic acid i.e. a beta-hydroxy acid that retards the rate of sebum production. Cleansing should be done twice a day (and considerably more in hot and humid situations) (and even more in hot and humid conditions).

Most of the oily skin care solutions are oil-free; nonetheless, it is always advisable to examine the contents of the product, before you really buy it. This is especially crucial if a product is labelled as 'suitable for all skin types', instead of 'oily skin care product'. 'Oily skin care' is also depending on the degree of oiliness, if you aren't too oily, therefore some of these 'suitable for all'- kind of products can be work for you too. For excessively oily skin, only oily skin care products are acceptable. Your oily skin care regimen might include an alcohol based toner (for an exceptionally oily skin) (for an extremely oily skin). This can be the second step in your oily skin care regimen i.e. shortly after cleansing.

However, excessive toning might hurt your skin.

The next step in your oily skin care routine might be a light moisturizer. Again, the degree of oiliness of your skin will determine if you need to include this in your oily skin care regimen. If you do decide to use a moisturizer, be sure to use one that is oil-free, wax-free and lipid-free.

You might also apply a clay mask (say once a week) as an oily skin care solution.

As far as the oily skin care products go, you might need to test out a few before you arrive at the one that is genuinely perfect for your skin.

In case these methods don't offer you the desired effect, see a qualified dermatologist for assistance. He might prescribe stronger oily skin care items like vitamin A creams, retinoids, sulphur creams etc , which can assist counter the issues of oily skin.

Tips For Make Up And Skin Care

'Make up and skin care' is often viewed as women's forte. Men seldom engage in 'Make up and skin care'. Many men do care for their skin but make up is extremely strange to most males.

Treating make up and skin care as independent issues wouldn't make sense; after all, make up will function only if the skin is healthy. So how can you exercise make up and skin care, together? Here are some recommendations for make up and skin care:

* Always have skin care on mind, whether you are buying goods for make up or actually applying them onto your skin once you have bought them. So what you are getting is a 'make up and skin care' product, not simply a make up product. Check the ingredients to determine whether it contains substances that you could be allergic to. Also

check whether it includes high concentration substances that might hurt your skin.

* 'Make up and skin care' is also about evaluating the goods before applying them. So, apply the make up on a small region of skin e.g. earlobes and evaluate how your skin reacts to it.

* Keep note of expiry date on your make up items and never use them past the expiry date. In reality certain items (e.g. vitamin C based products), if not stored properly, are ruined considerably sooner than the expiry date.

* Cleanliness is an important element of make up and skin care technique. Sharpen your eye-liners often and keep all your cosmetic tools clean at all times. You may designate a day, each month, for overhauling of your equipment. As part of hygiene, your make up and skin care

regimen should also involve keeping your hair clean at all times.

* Nail care is another crucial element of make up and skin care. Use an excellent quality nail polish and always keep your nails clean. Once you are done with washing and polishing your nails, you should rub in cuticle oil along the margins of the nail.

* If you have deep-set eyes, you should use a liquid eye liner instead of a pencil one. This will avoid smearing at the deep margins of your eye-lid.

* If you have a skin issue e.g. acne, you should not apply heavy or chemical based make up. Consult your dermatologist if you are not sure about the make up items that you can use when you have acne or other skin disease. Never try to squeeze pimples/ acne. Remember that make up and skin care should not contradict one other.

* Use a light make up remover (instead of just washing it away) (instead of just washing it away).

* Another vital 'make up and skin care' technique is the following golden rule: "Never sleep with your make up on"

* While applying a deodorant, make sure that you maintain the required distance between the nozzle and your skin (as specified on the deodorant box) (as mentioned on the deodorant pack).

So, make up and skin care should always go hand in hand. Do not try to approach make up and skin care differently.

Top 10 Skin Care Tips

Healthy skin is really one of the most significant factors for beauty-enhancement.

This post on skin care tips is an effort to deliver the 10 finest skin care ideas to you. The list of skin care recommendations has been reduced to 10 since anything more that that will not only be difficult to remember, but also shadow the most vital skin care suggestions. So let's see what these top 10 skin care suggestions are:

* Knowing your skin type is one of the most significant skin care advice. This is vital since not every skin care product suits everyone. In fact, all the skin care products identify the type of skin they cater too.

* 'Drink a lot of water'. This will not keep your skin moist but will aid in general care of your health (and in turn your skin) (and in turn your skin). It could seem a bit odd to some, but, this is a crucial skin care advice.

* Cleanse your skin frequently (1-2 times everyday) (1-2 times everyday). A highly powerful skin care technique that aids in getting rid of the dirt and other harsh elements from your skin. Cleansing is

especially vital after you have been out of your house (and consequently exposed to pollution, dust etc) (and hence exposed to pollutants, dust etc). This skin care advice also recommends the use of Luke warm water for cleaning (hot and cold water, both, do harm to your skin) (hot and cold water, both, cause damage to your skin)

* Be gentle, after all it's your skin. Don't scrub/exfoliate too hard or too often. Similarly, don't apply too much or too many skin care products. A must-to-follow skin care suggestion.

* Keep your skin moist at all times. This is one of the most significant skin care advice. Don't allow your skin grow dry. Dryness causes the surface layer of your skin to crack, leading to a harsh and unsightly look. Use moisturizers/ emollients. Moisturizers function best when applied when the skin is still wet.

* Avoid the use of soap on your face. Soap should only be used from below the neck. A modest yet vital skin care advice.

* Use sunscreen to protect yourself from sun's dangerous UV radiations. You can use day-time moisturizers that have sunscreen integrated into them. Use them even when it's overcast. UV radiations are known to cause skin cancer, therefore follow this skin care tip without fail.\s* A little of exercise and decent sleep are necessary too, not just for skin care but for your health as a whole.

Lack of sleep can lead to production of wrinkles underneath your eyes and lack of exercise might cause your skin to droop. Moreover, exercise and sleep also aid in overcoming stress. So aside being a skin care tip, this is also a health care tip.

* Treat skin issues with care. This skin care advice is about not neglecting any skin concerns. Consult your dermatologist before

you move on to utilize a skin care product (lest you do wind up hurting your skin even more) (lest you do end up harming your skin even more).

* Beat the tension. The detrimental effects of stress are known to everyone, but, sometimes stating the obvious is vital too (and therefore this skin care advice earned its way here) (and hence this skin care tip found its place here). Yes, stress damages skin too. So, take a break or indulge in a nice bubble bath or just get decent sleep.

Vitamin C Skin Care – The Challenge

Vitamin C is commonly recognized as a wrinkle fighter or an anti-aging agent. The basic purpose of 'Vitamin C skin care', in scientific words, is to enhance the synthesis of collagen (a structural protein that is found in skin) (a structural protein that is found in skin). The extra advantage of

'Vitamin C skin care' is connected to its potential of combating free radicals which cause harm to the skin.

Vitamin C skin care, however, confronts a serious issue nowadays. This is connected to the oxidation propensity of Vitamin C skin care products. On coming in touch with any oxidizing factor (e.g. air), the Vitamin C in the Vitamin C skin care products, is oxidized; therefore making the Vitamin C skin care product worthless (in fact counter-effective) (in fact counter-effective). The oxidized Vitamin C lends a yellowish-brown tint to the Vitamin C skin care product. This is something that you need to verify before choosing a Vitamin C skin care product. Even after you acquire a Vitamin C skin care product, you need to store it carefully and maintain ensuring that it's still okay to use (i.e. it hasn't obtained a yellowish-brown texture).

The makers of Vitamin C skin care products have tried to cope with this (oxidation) problem in many ways (and research on Vitamin C skin care products is on the top of their list) (and research on Vitamin C skin care products is on the top of their list). One such approach of keeping efficacy of Vitamin C skin care products for a long duration is to preserve a high concentration (say 10%) of Vitamin C. However, this makes the Vitamin C skin care products even more pricey. The Vitamin C skin care products are currently relatively affordable and making them much more expensive will push the product producers out of business. The alternative option is to employ Vitamin C derivatives (such ascorbyl palmitate and magnesium ascorbyl phosphate) (like ascorbyl palmitate and magnesium ascorbyl phosphate). These are not only more stable but also affordable. Even while the derivatives based products are not as effective as the Vitamin C skin care products, their durability against oxidation is a highly desired property that makes them very popular. Moreover, they are reported to be less annoying too.

Talking of effectiveness of Vitamin C skin care products, it's necessary to emphasize that not everyone reacts to Vitamin C therapies. So it's not a magic potion in any manner. If you don't observe a visible improvement in your skin, it may be due of your skin not reacting to Vitamin C therapy (and the Vitamin C skin care products might not be at blame, at all) (and the Vitamin C skin care products might not be at fault, at all).

As further study goes on, one can only keep our fingers crossed and wait for a comprehensive answer to the issues encountered by 'Vitamin C skin care' today.

What Is Natural Skin Care?

Put simply, 'natural skin care' involves caring for your skin in a natural and chemical-free method. 'Natural skin care' encourages permitting the skin to take care of itself (without any aid from synthetic materials/ chemicals). 'Natural skin care' is about inculcation of beneficial habits in the way you run your day to day life. A lot of natural skin care methods are essentially the same as those for body care in general.

So let's explore what these natural skin care measures are.

Well the first and the primary natural skin care measure is – 'Drink a lot of water'. Around 8 glasses of water is a necessary everyday. Water aids in cleaning out the toxins from the body, in a natural way. It assists in the general care of the body and supports excellent health for all organs (not just skin) (not just skin).

General cleaning is another affordable technique of natural skin care. Daily shower, wearing clean clothing and sleeping on a clean mattress/pillow are all part of overall cleanliness. After all, clean skin is the key to keeping the skin problems at bay.

Regular exercise is the next thing on the cards. Exercise boosts the flow of blood that aids in getting rid of bodily toxins and keeping you healthy. Exercise also helps in overcoming stress which is the deadliest enemy of good health.

Healthy food and eating habits are also suggested for natural skin care. Some sort of food (e.g. greasy food) is know to induce acne and should be avoided as much as possible. Your diet should be a balanced mix of diverse nutrition supplying items. Raw fruits and vegetables are believed to bring freshness to your body and aid in getting rid of bodily toxins.

A decent sleep is also crucial in sustaining good health and in conquering stress. As a natural skin care measure, a healthy sleep avoids sagging of skin.

Beating stress is another natural skin care therapy. Stress causes general harm to body and health. Drinking a lot of water, getting a great sleep and exercising has previously been recommended as stress busters. Indulging in a nice bubble bath, listening to music and playing your favorite

sport are also wonderful techniques of combating stress. Yoga is yet another means of overcoming stress; it is swiftly gaining favor amongst the population.

Avoiding excessive exposure to sun (by wearing long sleeved garments, hat and umbrella etc), is another natural skin care method. Sunscreen creams are also advised if necessary.

A lot of traditional and home manufactured natural skin care products/ methods are also proven to be quite effective. Such steps are not only natural and easy-to-follow, but also reasonably affordable.

Besides that, a variety of natural skin care products are accessible in the commercial sector. These include products like lavender oil, aloe Vera etc., which don't have any adverse effects.

Which Is The Best Skin Care Product?

There is truly nothing like a great skin care product. There truly can't be something like 'The greatest skin care product', because skin care products perform differently for various people (depending on the skin type to some extent) (based on the skin type to some extent). A product that is the 'best skin care product' for one person could wind up being the worst for another person. So, a more natural question to ask would be 'What is the best skin care product for my kind of skin?' However, this still is not totally reasonable. We prefer to split people into 4 groups depending on their skin characteristics – i.e. dry skin, oily skin, normal skin and sensitive skin.

However, this categorization is just too wide to be utilized decisively in identifying the finest skin care product. We may say 'best skin care product for a dry skin' or 'best skin care product for an oily skin' are better assertions than merely 'best skin care product'. But really, that is what it is – 'better'; still not accurate.

So, it really comes to rephrasing the question to – 'What is the best skin care product for me'. Yes, this is precisely the issue that you should be asking, and sadly there is no easy solution for this. Arriving at the ideal skin care product for self will take some work on your behalf.

First of all, you need to understand how the skin care products function. This is simple. You may consider all skin care products to be constituted of 2 categories of substances - Active and inactive. The active chemicals are the ones that truly function on your skin. The inactive ones only aid in delivering these active substances to your skin. Both the components need to work for your skin, in order for the product to be successful (and progress on to become the greatest skin care product for you) (and move on to become the best skin care product for you).

Besides the contents, the method you apply your skin care products is as significant. In reality, this is far more vital. If you do not know how to apply skin care products, you might forever be hunting for the best skin care product for yourself, when that has already passed you. Moreover, it's also important to decide on the frequency of application (of the skin care product) (of the skin care product). The environmental conditions - temperature, humidity and pollution level, also impact the choosing of finest skin care product. Here are a few principles that you might utilize to guarantee that your best skin care product is indeed the best for you:

* Cleanse your skin before applying that best skin care product.\s* Use a makeup remover instead of plain water and remove your makeup before going to bed.

* The efficiency of active substances is diminished when put over another product e.g. over moisturizer. So use the best skin care product first and then add a dab of moisturizer if needed.

* Apply the items on damp and heated skin.

* You will have to experiment with a few products before you arrive at the one that is the best skin care product for you.\s* Do not exfoliate too much or too hard.\s* Vary your skin care routine as per the seasons (winter/summer etc), changes in environmental factors and changes in your skin type

Note that the optimum skin care product cannot be established overnight. It's only through trial (and knowledge) that you can locate the 'Best skin care product' (for you) (for you).

Reducing Wrinkles: Is There A Way?

Reducing wrinkles is something that many of use look forward to accomplishing. As the body ages, so does the skin. The sun, our food and merely our genetic DNA have a part in exactly how much we have to struggle with this illness. One thing is for sure. If you don't want to appear your age, wrinkles are something that should be on your mind. Engraved in the thoughts of all of us is that concept that if we have wrinkles, that it is a symptom of becoming old. Yet, remember that wrinkles can emerge at nearly any period during your life. That implies, you may look older than you feel or truly are.

One of the most significant things for you to perform in order to confront the well being of your skin is to be informed about it. Start by having a look at what a wrinkle truly is. It is a ridge where the skin is no longer flat. Fine wrinkles only appear like little lines but they are the early stages of much more dramatic looking wrinkles. The folds of your skin, which is what wrinkles truly are, might appear for a number of reasons. In theory, they are due to the skin becoming more elastic and the tissue underneath the skin becoming too loose or even removed partially.

Why did you have to get wrinkles? Most of the time, wrinkles are a part of everyone's aging process. The skin gets looser as a result of losing collagen below. When it happens, the skin will fold naturally with gravity. For some, the significant quantity of wrinkles that they have might be related to over exposure to the sun, to a lack of a nutritious diet and even to hereditary causes.

Is there something that you can do about these conditions? There are. In reality, there are several things that you can do. Start with providing yourself the nutrition that your body needs to keep your skin looking wonderful. There are over the counter remedies for wrinkles, too. Some of these function, while others do not. You can resort to plastic surgery or to chemical injections to restore the missing collagen. There are a variety of techniques to improve the look of your face and skin.

5 Tips for Reducing Wrinkles

Reducing wrinkles is something most will want to tackle at some point. Many people do not realize they are aging until they look in the mirror for the first time and notice wrinkles.Sure, it took a very long time for them to get there, but it doesn't imply that you saw this coming. What's more is that for many, wrinkles are going to happen no matter what you do. It's in your DNA! These realities are not often grasped, though. And, when you want to find a remedy that will help you to genuinely reduce the wrinkles on your face, consider these items.

1. Eat the right foods.Fill your day with dark green veggies, bright reds, orange tones, and more. Consuming these goods will provide your body with the nutrition and the antioxidants it needs to keep your blood moving. This helps to keep your skin moisturized and fends against wrinkles.

2. Wear sun protection every time you come into contact with the sun.Even in the winter or on gloomy days, the UV rays come through and your skin needs protection. The sun is the #1 causative agent of early wrinkles.

3. Exfoliate. If you enable your skin to have a fresh start every week, then it will always seem young. There are several lotions and washes that may be utilized to give this support to you, too. It might be as simple as washing your face with them.

4. When evaluating wrinkle creams, opt for ones that include Vitamin A, Vitamin C, and Vitamin E in them. These are fantastic for aiding in fighting off wrinkles and restoring life to your skin again.

5. Remove make-up and excess oils from your face on a regular basis.If you don't allow your skin the health that it requires, you will find yourself having problems with

wrinkles. Don't dry out your skin, either, though. Removing the gunk from your pores is necessary for good-looking skin and fewer wrinkles.

Although there are no products that can promise that they will help you to eradicate the wrinkles on your face and neck, there are numerous methods by which you may improve the skin quality that you have. If you search for a high-quality product and maintain excellent health standards, the final effect is a better-looking you.

Can Diet Help Reduce Wrinkles?

When it comes to eating a healthy diet, experts will tell you that most Americans just don't get it. Yet, if you are aging, now is the most critical moment in your life to start thinking about this topic. What you consume has a major impact on the healthy glow that you have. If you don't eat healthily, you are more prone to having to deal with dreadful wrinkles. If you would like to see fewer wrinkles, one of the best things for you to do is to eat a well-balanced diet.

There are several things that have a part in the wellness of your body. While bacteria and genetics do play a role to some degree in your wrinkles, it is not all that impacts them. In truth, many women and men will acquire wrinkles much before their age determines it to be required. This has a lot to do with the nutritious nutrition that you are probably not receiving.

Diet? Dieting for Wrinkles?

How might your food genuinely affect your wrinkles? First and foremost, recognize that wrinkles may be created by a variety of causes, including the inability of the body to maintain hold of a material called collagen. When your body loses this, your skin will get looser and that contributes to wrinkles. If you feed your body the correct nutrition to get through these conditions, you can actually walk away with fewer wrinkles and enhanced skin care.

One thing to consider eating is more veggies. Vegetables include antioxidants, which are true soldiers in battling numerous health hazards. These substances go into your bloodstream and essentially clean up the cells. By doing this, they allow blood to readily move through the body.
When it happens, your skin looks fantastic and plump. In reality, antioxidants play a significant part in minimizing your wrinkles
.

What should you eat? To decrease the wrinkles that you now have or to help prevent even more from popping up, take a diet that is high in antioxidants. Eat a diet that is balanced with fresh vegetables, lean proteins, and unsaturated fats. These elements will lead to a healthy diet that delivers numerous benefits to your general well-being. When you give your body the tools that it needs, it will be better equipped to minimize wrinkles and give you radiant, attractive skin.

Reducing Wrinkles: Over The Counter Wrinkle Cream

When it comes to minimizing wrinkles, there are a lot of different over-the-counter cream solutions that you might utilize. Many times, these are marketed to you as a miraculous treatment for your wrinkles, allowing you to easily apply the cream and watch the wrinkles go away. Do you know exactly how virtually impossible that is? It didn't take your skin only a few days to generate those wrinkles, and it is likely to take more than a few days to get rid of them, too. Before you write off these creams as something that just doesn't work, examine how they can genuinely work for you.

Some over-the-counter wrinkle treatments have proven some help in decreasing wrinkles, but not all do. If you want to use this strategy to combat your wrinkles, then make sure that the product that you purchase contains the following substances, which have been linked to enhancing the condition of your skin. While all of these components haven't been investigated sufficiently to provide you with full assurance, they tend to be the most effective at combating wrinkles and restoring a healthy look to the face.

•Vitamin A: This antioxidant has been one of the forerunners in decreasing wrinkles. Look for skin creams and wrinkle reducers that have this in them, but make sure that it is as high of an amount as possible. This vitamin helps to break down free radicals, which cause your skin cells to break down.

• Hydroxy Acids: Consider this exfoliating product.You want a wrinkle cream that will offer this since it will eliminate the top layers of dead skin and allow your skin to generate new skin that is healthy looking.

• Alpha Lipoic Acid: An antioxidant that can penetrate cell membranes.When it does this, it helps to get rid of free radicals that break down the cells in your skin. This also works effectively at enhancing the efficacy of other antioxidants that accomplish the same task. Vitamin C and Vitamin E are fantastic choices.

If you are wanting to decrease wrinkles with the use of over-the-counter creams, skin lotions, and agents, then choose just those that have a good number of these ingredients in them. They have proved to be the most useful for improving the look of the skin and eliminating the appearance of wrinkles all together.

Reducing Wrinkles: Understanding Botox

To decrease wrinkles, consider Botox. Many individuals are looking for a remedy that will assist them to get rid of the wrinkles that have been creeping up on them over the course of a lifetime.

Although most individuals do not understand that with proper skin care and a balanced diet they may minimize the number of wrinkles they have, many are considering chemical injections such as Botox. If you are wondering about it, examine these facts about Botox and others like it first.

What is it?

Botox is delivered by injections straight into the skin's deep layers. There, it assists by relaxing the face muscles that are around your wrinkles. This makes them much less obvious. Because the muscles are relaxed, the skin lies smoother, allowing for fewer obvious wrinkles there. The actual chemical that is injected is botulinum toxin type A, which is a refined and harmless form of the toxin that causes botulism. The injections are not all that unpleasant and are typically regarded as a quick remedy to the problem of wrinkles. Yet, is this the appropriate decision for you?

Where Can You Use It?

Botox may be applied in numerous ways and will have the same effect in each region that it is used in. The most common sites for them are around the corners of the eyes, the frown lines that run between your eyebrows and the bridge of your nose, your forehead, and the wrinkle bands in the neck area.

What you should know is that Botox won't work if your wrinkles have been created by sun exposure. It also doesn't work on all the wrinkles on your face. Also, for some, the thickness of the skin and the type of skin that you have will impact how successful Botox will be for you.

Is Botox the right thing for you? To find out if you qualify and if, in fact, it might be good for your wrinkles, consider talking to an expert.

Remember that Botox is not a cure and that you will need to continue having the procedure done to keep the wrinkles at bay. Over time, it may not be as helpful for you if additional wrinkles emerge. Nonetheless, many women are discovering that Botox is the ideal solution to their desire to remove wrinkles.

Reducing Wrinkles: Using Home Remedies

Did you believe you might reduce your wrinkles with the help of some really decent home remedies? The reality is that there are numerous things that you have sitting around your home that might be good for your health. Some of these cures have been passed down for thousands of years. Why have they endured so long? Maybe because of precisely how useful they can be.

While there is no actual means of getting rid of all the wrinkles that you have, several of these products can give you a wide variety of advantages, helping to avoid wrinkles from deepening and preventing them from being extremely obvious.

Here are a few terrific methods for getting rid of wrinkles with the use of home remedies.

1. Schedule a massage.When you receive a decent massage, your body is going to feel wonderful, but it is also going to look beautiful. A massage will really accelerate the circulation moving through your body, helping to clear out and rebuild cells faster and more efficiently. Your muscles are looser, too, helping to ease those wrinkles.

2. Apply a solution of turmeric powder and sugarcane juice (one part turmeric powder to one part sugarcane juice) to your

wrinkles.Apply it to your wrinkled areas regularly to observe the benefits.

3. Green Thompson seedless grapes can also be useful. Squeeze them and apply the juice to your face. Let it rest for about twenty minutes and rinse.

4. Apply the juice of green pineapples to your face every day.Leave it in place for at least 10 minutes. This can also assist in eliminating broken skin that you may have.

5. For finer lines, put the core of a pineapple on your skin. Keep it in the sink for at least 10 minutes and then rinse with warm water. This will help to get rid of some of those fine creases that you know will end up being bigger ones.

Home treatments that can help decrease wrinkles are harmless unless you are sensitive to the substance. There are hundreds of other possibilities out there as well. If you are interested in discovering the greatest home remedies for your skin care requirements, take a glance into your pantry and forget about the pricey skin care regimens that are available.

Reducing Wrinkles: Using Laser Resurfacing

When it comes to the wrinkles that you have, whether you want to accept them or not, you have to do something about them. You may have those small wrinkles forming under your eyes. Or, you may be staring at the laugh lines that just don't appear at all amusing any more. Wrinkles are a genuine indicator that you are aging. But, remember, you are only as youthful as you feel. With that in mind, consider how laser resurfacing could be the treatment that you are after to reduce the signs of aging that are creeping up on you.

First off, what is it? Laser resurfacing is precisely what it sounds like. With the use of a laser, your old, damaged, and aged skin is eliminated. This helps your body to naturally develop new skin that is healthier, younger looking, and with fewer apparent wrinkles. In all reality, nothing can totally eliminate every wrinkle on your face. However, laser resurfacing has been shown to be quite potentially beneficial to many people.

Laser resurfacing will genuinely work in a lot of circumstances. It is particularly effective on the fine wrinkles of your skin, but it works on moderate wrinkles too. It can also help with other aging symptoms like liver spots and age spots.If you have skin that has been harmed by the ever pounding sun, that too can be treated. Did you experience a lot of acne growing up that left you with scars? All of these items can possibly be helped with the use of laser resurfacing.

The method is not that tough.

You will face a tiny light energy laser that will very rapidly and efficiently destroy the very top layer of skin on the places that are to be treated. It will then heat the underlying skin, called the dermis, enough that it will promote the skin to grow. Because it has removed the top layer of skin, your body will need to replace the region with new skin.

The skin that comes in will be healthy and will have fewer obvious wrinkles.
Is laser resurfacing the appropriate therapy for your wrinkles? Many have utilized it and experienced amazing success. The greatest potential answer for you is to select the most qualified specialist to conduct the task for you, since skill plays a great deal of a part in the quality of the operation.
Reducing Wrinkles: Do Over-The-Counter Remedies Work?

There are hundreds of products on the market that promise to be able to provide you with a wide range of wrinkle reduction features. If you stroll into a department shop and take a look at the items, you are likely to encounter an entire section that is just full of wrinkle creams of one form or another. Do they work? If you question the salesperson, they will most likely tell you about some magical product that they used.Really, though, there are a lot of aspects that play a role in simply whether the product will function. The main fact, though, is that not all wrinkle reduction products do.

It is up to you to locate those that do function, though. To assist you, here are a number of ideas to allow you to locate the best potential answer to your wrinkle problems.

1. Take a look at the components. If you are shopping on the web or you are purchasing

locally, have a look at the ingredients. Sure, there are terms you don't know there. But, you should be able to notice a number of important vitamins present. Vitamin A is the most crucial as it is one of the best wrinkle fighters out there. Look for Vitamin C and Vitamin E, too.

2. Browse the internet for a while.There is more product potential on the web than any business can supply. What's more is that the name brand is absolutely s3. There is no indication of the quality of the goods. In fact, it may not be one that works well for you at all, but another generic would. Keep your choices open here.

4. Anticipate what others will say to you.Wrinkle creams are not affordable, and for that reason, you need the guidance and expert opinion of others. Make sure that you are comparing their conditions to your own and see if they match. Also, consider that they may or may not have used the product

as it was advised. Nevertheless, internet evaluations of numerous wrinkle reduction solutions can enable you to make a choice.

You deserve quality, and for that reason, you should pick wrinkle creams that can deliver it to you. The reality is that there are many that can bring benefits, but just as many, if not more, that are leading you on.

Reducing Wrinkles: Start With Prevention

When it comes to wrinkles, there are various reasons why you may acquire them. But, the reality is that you will continue to acquire more and they can even deepen if you don't make efforts early on to stop them. There are various sorts of wrinkle products on the market. Home cures and cosmetic operations might help you to lessen the wrinkles that you have, too. But, before you go through with it, you should understand that there are also a number of other options accessible to you to aid you in avoiding even more wrinkles from cropping up.

How to Prevent Wrinkles

Stay out of the sun. Using sunscreen whenever you go outside doesn't sound like fun, but it is, in fact, the best way to keep age spots and wrinkles at bay. Although most people may not understand it, the sun is one of the worst things that you could experience for your skin. It takes away the moisture and the UV radiation can create far more serious diseases than just wrinkles, including skin cancers.

• Establish a daily routine.Having a decent quality washing program will also assist in keeping your skin healthy and shining rather than aching and uncomfortable. There are a lot of ways to achieve this, but you want to be sure of several crucial factors. First, pick a cleanser that can remove make-up and oils from your skin without drying it out. If you have dry skin, opt for a moisturizer. You also want to integrate an exfoliating product into your regimen as this will aid in eliminating the top layers of dead skin cells and allow for a more appealing look.

Eat a diet high in antioxidants. This will even enable you to eliminate the creases that you currently have. A diet that is rich in healthy veggies is the best place to start. Look for deep-colored veggies for the absolute best outcomes. Antioxidants function to eliminate free radicals, which are like trash that clogs up your blood flow and your cells. Removing them helps to keep your skin healthy.

Reducing wrinkles is a requirement. Those who are seeking a solution to reap the benefits of good skin and a decrease in wrinkles need to focus on not just erasing

what they have but also preventing additional wrinkles from taking shape.
Reducing Wrinkles Through A Facelift

Are you wondering precisely how you might boost the condition of your skin? Are you attempting to learn precisely how you can get rid of the age lines that life has given you? You may then be considering a facelift. A facelift is not as dramatic as it seems, but it is still an elective procedure that does have certain complication risk factors like other operations do. Is this the best therapy for you?

What is it?

A facelift is a type of surgery that has the ability to achieve various things for you. First, it will help tighten loose skin on your face and neck. This allows you to get rid of the wrinkles that are there. A facelift is radical enough to help even some of the worst wrinkles seem significantly less obvious, if not eradicate them. It is excellent for the area around the nose and the lips, as well as helping to eliminate the fat from the neck area. If you are concerned about your body's capacity to look young, here is one technique to tackle it.

There are numerous sorts of facelifts that are accessible. For example, the tiniest are termed "feather lifts," which will require very little invasive surgery to help erase a few wrinkles in the appropriate spot. More in-depth coverage is that of the deep plane lifts, which will aid in tightening huge muscle groups in contrast. When you undergo a facelift, you may even wish to consider implants. These can be implanted in your cheekbones, in your jaw or in other locations to help define your skin's inherent attractiveness and eliminate the wrinkles there.

When it comes to the cost of a facelift, there are various variances. There are various aspects that have a part in that decision. For example, the expertise and reputation of your doctor will influence the cost.Various parts of the country also provide distinct pricing tiers, with the most costly locations being those of California and New York. In addition, the sort of operation that you have done will also impact the amount of the expense.

Is a facelift the right option for you? Many people have had this process done and have walked out of the doctor's office looking 10, 20, or more years younger with the decrease of wrinkles.

Anti-Aging: Can You Defy The Odds?

"Anti-aging" is a word that is used widely today. Yet, there are various methods in which you might notice a healthier skin or enhanced health and even defy the chances of getting older. As your body ages, each aspect of it seems to perform less properly, and that's where the trouble typically resides. But, if you can successfully manage to cater to the demands that your body is currently lacking, you may really be able to effectively obtain the rewards that you are seeking and at least look as youthful as you feel.

Anti-aging choices are plentiful; that's the first thing that you will find when you do a quick search for them. But, before you do that, and have yourself assaulted with many spam emails that seem to give no actual advantage, look at what it is that your body is needing. Often, it is only a matter of catering to the new demands your body has.

When you were born, your parents gave you the highest quality nutrients so that your body could grow. Later, when you were a young adult, you learned how to eat in the appropriate manner and do the things required to maintain your weight. As you age, you need to recognize your body's changing demands and prepare for them. That's the trick.

What does your body require that you are not providing for? If you are aging, one of the first things to consider is calcium for healthy bones. Without extra calcium, your body's requirements still grow and to receive the calcium that is necessary, it must go to your bones to get it. That weakens bones, causes discomfort and can possibly lead to more damage. But, what about anti-aging for the skin?

The skin ages in its own manner. The body doesn't manufacture the collagen that it used to, which causes your wrinkles to form. There is simply just not enough fat under the skin to allow the skin to stand up. To fix this condition, simply invest in a nutritious diet filled with antioxidants. Or, you can go for injections and cosmetic touch-ups that can assist in restoring some of the lost collagen.

Finding out what your body requires and then adding additional resources to it to assist in supplying those requirements is a terrific method to avoid aging and defy the odds. You may boost your body's potential to defy aging by caring for your needs now, while you still have the power to do so.

Cosmetic Surgeons For Anti-Aging: How To Choose

There are a lot of factors to consider when it comes to anti-aging. It starts with determining if cosmetic surgery is right for you. If so, and it is the correct option for many, it's crucial to take your time and choose the best surgeon for the process. If you don't engage in this procedure, you might find yourself needing to have numerous surgeries when it could have only taken one. Cosmetic surgeons appear to improve with experience. With greater experience, they are more confident and precise. These are things you absolutely want to avoid when it comes to your cosmetic demands for anti-aging remedies.

How to Find the Right Doctor

Before you step into the doctor's office, do your homework at home first. The first thing to do is to learn about the doctor's record. You can do this by looking them up online, using the Better Business Bureau, contacting your local regulatory services, or simply looking for individual evaluations directly online.You are likely to locate other patients who have worked with him as well as those who have a personal history with various features of that doctor. The aim is to understand if he or she has the experience that is favorable for your needs.

Next, schedule a consultation with the doctor to discuss your cosmetic surgery. Go with your interests here. If you don't like them, can't comprehend what they are saying to you or discover that they are not satisfying your requirements by addressing what is vital to you, then don't utilize them. Most consultations are question and answer sessions, which will help you choose the individual who is most credible to you. This is also a fantastic chance to ask questions about the past and to see before and after images of things that they've personally done as well. Will they allow you to communicate with other patients? Do they answer your inquiries clearly? The final line here is if you like and trust the doctor. If you do, then proceed.

Getting some more information and research on your doctor is a vital factor. It will help you to feel good about the person whom you are placing your life and appearance in the hands of. With a few extra minutes of completing these things, you are likely to feel better about the whole procedure and even obtain the benefits of superior anti-aging remedies.
Consider Anti-Aging Techniques Carefully.

Did you know that the market for anti-aging goods will reach well over 42 billion dollars this year? The trouble with a market that is so vast is that many times there are items and needs that just don't mesh with those that do work. As individuals and organizations realize the rising expectations that customers have, they are more inclined than ever to enhance their products so that they too may obtain a portion of that money. Yet, many times, their items are not worth the amount that you'll pay for them. In that sense, you need to pay attention and complete your homework.

Why It Matters

On the market at any one time, there are thousands of products claiming to be the next great thing for anti-aging. Some individuals discover that there are components that demand their attention more so than others. When it comes to selecting anti-aging products, you need to take care.

Here are some recommendations to enable you to make the proper choices regarding the anti-aging goods you purchase and utilize.

1. Complete your homework.Take the time to research the firm that manufactures the goods. You may do this straight online at the Better Business Bureau's website. Find out what sort of difficulties they have, if any, so that you don't make the same mistakes that others do.

2.Look for information from other users. Often times, you may uncover reviews on things that might actually meet your needs. Take a look at the sorts of items offered and then hunt for reviews of them. Find out what others have found out about those items. Are they truly worth the cost?

3. Determine why they work.Just because something contains natural substances in it

does not indicate that it is going to provide you with fewer wrinkles. Find out if the science behind it truly does make sense. A product that can't deliver this for you is one that you should avoid.

There is no doubt that you need to devote a few more minutes to choosing the correct anti-aging solutions for your needs. In many circumstances, taking extra time will pay off as you will have the very greatest items and the best overall investment that you can make.

Using Calorie Restriction

One type of anti-aging procedure that seems to be highly successful is that of limiting the quantity of calories that are ingested. This hypothesis is one that is not entirely understood, by any means, but it is something that should be carefully explored regardless. Why does calorie restriction help the body lose weight? The proof of it happening is evident, but why it happens, most physicians are not too sure. Nevertheless, it is a fantastic solution for folks seeking a strategy to fight aging indications throughout their body.

What Is Likely Happening?

Calorie restriction helps to postpone illness as well as live a longer life. The concept behind this sort of anti-aging remedy is that by limiting the quantity of calories you consume, you will also lessen the amount of insulin that your body creates. With this decrease in insulin, the signs of aging will be reduced. That's because insulin is also an accelerant of the aging process.

With decreased calories, we observe advantages because of the lower oxidative stressors from those calories as well. You've heard of the advantages of antioxidants. By consuming meals in a less hurried fashion, there is less "bad" coming in with the potential of more beneficial antioxidants going in. This may also allow you to improve your overall health.

For calorie restriction to work for you, though, you need to engage with your dietician and understand what foods are must-haves and which should be avoided. You aren't going to necessarily take out everything, but every calorie must count in this approach, instead of allowing empty calories into your diet. You also need to avoid meal replacement solutions, as these rarely deliver the same advantages as proper, nutritious nourishment. You may even find out which foods are regarded as super foods in that they contain great amounts of nutrients with decent levels of calories.

If you do pick a calorie restriction approach to anti-aging, go for it with the help and guidance of your doctor. You should look at what you are eating and not try to merely cut back on how much you are eating. The objective here is not to starve yourself in any manner. Instead, it is to replace the high-calorie, poor-meals in your diet with items that are deemed very healthy with lower calorie counts.

Anti-Aging And Cosmetic Surgery

There is no question that one of the most effective ways for folks to acquire anti-aging aid is to employ cosmetic surgery. The term "cosmetic" is used to indicate something that is done to fix the look of something rather than the function of it. Perhaps with cosmetic surgery, though, the objective is more than simply restoring the way that your skin appears but also the way that you feel about yourself. If you believe that your wrinkles are bringing down your self-esteem, it might be highly advantageous to your well-being to engage in any sort of cosmetic surgery.

What is spent
Currently, the cosmetic surgery market is rising by leaps and bonds. Each year there is an increase of extreme proportions in the number of operations done. Both men and women will endure these processes. In

addition, there is no doubt that the cost of doing so will climb from $20 billion in 2003 to well over $50 billion by 2007, or more. The most popular age group that undergoes cosmetic surgery is that of 35 to 50. But, is this a terrible thing?

Is it bad?
There can't be anyone that argues that cosmetic surgery is certainly negative, unless it puts you at danger from other health concerns that you may have. But, there are hazards associated with Without a qualified surgeon, you may have to have more than one treatment done. There are usually a handful of surgical mishaps each year, too. In addition, there is nothing cheap or affordable when it comes to this anti-aging remedy.

But, cosmetic surgery does increase self-confidence, which many physicians and scientists feel may aid an individual to improve their health across the board. If you are favorably motivated, you can do more physically and psychologically. If you are sad, sickness and disease set in much more so. For this reason, there are health advantages to cosmetic surgery that will improve the outlook that the patient has.

Is cosmetic surgery for you? Weighing the expenses, the hazards, and the total reward can only be done by you. If you do go down this road, you will need to invest in studying to locate the finest specialist for your treatment. In the appropriate hands, dangers are minimized and processes are more successful.

A Good Diet For Anti-Ageing Benefits

No matter if you like to hear it or not, a decent, balanced diet is one of the best weapons for anti-aging advantages. The basis is basic. If you provide your body with the nutrition and the correct fuel that it requires, you will receive optimum outcomes from it. Consider your automobile, for example. If you don't give it the proper sort of gasoline, it will wear down faster, won't perform nearly as well, won't get the right gas mileage, and it probably won't last as long. If you give it the maximum possible fuel, on the other hand, you'll see that it runs longer, better, and has fewer troubles along the road.

This same thing works for your body. Your body requires all of the proper nutrients if it is to accomplish the things that you want it to do and to deliver the right amount of anti-aging capabilities. Many people make the error of seeking another approach to enhance their situation rather than looking at their own specific requirements. Rather than working for greater health through an effective approach, such as through a balanced diet, they search for other answers that may be simpler to make happen. Yet, there is simply nothing more effective than monitoring what you consume for your body's wellness.

What Your Body Requires:

For your body to have a balanced diet, it requires a high level of nutrients and a low level of saturated fats and carbohydrates. For example, you need veggies. Most vegetables include significant amounts of nutrients and also provide a good number of antioxidants, which help stimulate cells, enhance blood circulation, and eliminate toxins from the body.

That in and of itself is an achievement that you require in regards to enhancing your aging. A wonderful method to incorporate more of them into your diet is through vegetable juices. Replace your sodas with veggie drinks (prepare them yourself for increased nutrition and cheaper prices!)

You should also remove from your diet anything that might cause potential difficulties. For example, sugars are a concern since they help manufacture insulin. Insulin is an aging accelerant and is something you don't need extra of. By lowering the quantity of sugar you eat, you reduce the amount of insulin, which therefore lowers the aging effects it will have on your body.

Simply by considering how you can improve your diet, you can obtain some of the most effective anti-aging treatments available.

Exercise And Anti-Aging

Exercise is often considered a positive thing, but when it comes to anti-aging needs, it may be something you need to manage. By far, you must include some sort of exercise in your normal day. Yet, you shouldn't incorporate too much exercise either. This restriction is one that many people that are starting to feel those aging indications need to pay greater attention to. With a few guiding tools, you can efficiently manage the aging requirements that you have.

Regular Exercise Is A Must

Make no mistake, you need to acquire regular exercise. By moving your body, you use the fuel that you have placed in it. You keep it moving; keep it burning that fuel so that it doesn't add extra pounds to your belly or elsewhere on your body. Weight gain can be dangerous to one's overall health, causing a person to age faster than he or she needs to.By lowering your weight, you can really boost your health tenfold.
manage to accomplish this and progress is around the corner.

Too Much Isn't A Good Thing.

But, when it comes to anti-aging demands that you may have, you should take into account the fact that too much, or excessive, exercise is not such a wonderful thing for you. Many experts feel that extreme activity, such as running a marathon every weekend, might do damage to your skin. Here, the concern comes with too much cardiovascular and aerobic activity. If you perform this sort of activity and don't provide your body with the necessary levels of antioxidants that are required, you will rapidly find yourself suffering with damaged skin.

Your body has various demands and one of them is for the correct quantity of antioxidants to assist in eliminating pollutants and prevent oxidative damage to your body. If you exercise at a high level, you cause more oxidative damage to your skin as part of the process. Remember that excessive activity stresses several regions of the body, including the skin.

Without filling those needs with increased levels of antioxidants (even with large amounts of additional antioxidants in your diet), your skin would age quicker than it would if you only had a normal quantity of exercise. While receiving this degree of activity is appropriate provided you do provide the correct antioxidant protection, lowering the stress of it on your body can enhance your aging.

Do Anti-Aging Products Work?

You go through the aisles of your favorite department store and notice various anti-aging products. They reach out to you with promises of making you look the best you have since you were a teenager. Many make claims that are everything but practical, and, regrettably, many of them won't work for you. However, there are many that can provide exactly what you are looking for: better skin, healthy-looking skin, and youthful-looking skin.It can happen, and there are several solutions to explore.

Learning What Works

The main issue you must struggle through is discovering which items are beneficial and which are not even potentially so. Here are some pointers to knowing which the greatest anti-aging products on the market are.

1. Expand your knowledge.Find out why they function. What is their pledge to you? Does it make scientific sense to work? Finding out not only what they promise to accomplish but why they work may frequently remove those that don't make sense or those that may not be suited for you.

2. Learn from those who are knowledgeable.Others have more than likely utilized the anti-aging product in the past. Take the necessary time to discover what their experiences have been. Find out if they would recommend them to others, or maybe not. You can do this quickly and easily on the internet.

3. Research the firm.Companies who repeatedly put items on the market that offer little advantage to most consumers commonly complain to the Better Business Bureau. You may also look into the firm and its products more completely through the Consumer Reports website. Either of these options will provide you with more information about whether this company is genuine in their claims of anti-aging products that work.

Follow the directions

Another typical difficulty that people that use anti-aging products find is that they don't function. But, this happens not because the product doesn't have the ability to operate, but rather that they did not use it effectively. That provides for the worst possible circumstance. Following the guidelines provided will undoubtedly boost your body's capacity to gain maximum advantage from the product.

Anti-aging items that are thoroughly studied and are used as they are meant to be used are products that may provide a lot of aid and well-being to an individual. They can provide you with advantages in terms of improved health and wellness.

A Great Anti-Aging Technique: Get Enough Sleep!

Do you get enough sleep? If you are seeking an anti-aging strategy that will work for you, make sure you still get enough sleep in the process. There is no doubt that your body is going to age as the years go by. But, the quantity of aging that is experienced in your physical appearance and health is something that may be managed to some degree. No matter what method you take to enhance your general health and decrease the indications of aging, be sure that sleep is part of the package.

Sleep Is Required.

Sleeping is your body's way of mending and improving. When you sleep, your body uses your energy and resources to enhance your health, to repair cells, to develop and even to improve your health. For that reason, it is crucial in the anti-aging process to evaluate if you receive enough sleep to allow your body to accomplish what it has to do to preserve your health and also your skin's beauty.

Can You Get Enough?

Doctors will suggest that individuals require at least eight hours of sleep every night. Your body may require more or less, as each person is different. The method to tell if you are getting enough sleep is straightforward. Do you wake up in the morning feeling refreshed? Or, are you exhausted and starting your day hoping you could sleep for a few more minutes? Without enough sleep, your body can't do what it is necessary to do. So, attempt to find techniques to improve your sleep. Here are some strategies that may help you get to sleep quickly.

• Avoid eating meals or even heavily sugared snacks at least two hours before night since they will boost your blood sugar and keep you awake.

• Listen to white noise (natural noise) or relaxation CDs.Getting in some meditation before bed helps as well.

Don't watch television before bed. Television stimulates your intellect, which keeps you attentive and thinking. Instead, choose a calming hobby to do.

Adequate sleep is essential for people who use anti-aging therapies or simply want to improve their overall health.Find out what it can do for you by getting to bed sooner and truly getting the sleep your body demands. It might be the perfect companion to other anti-aging therapies too.

Cosmetic Surgery Considerations For Anti-Aging

If you are contemplating cosmetic surgery for the greatest potential anti-aging treatments for your needs, evaluate precisely who you are looking for. There are various factors that you should bear in mind when it comes to enhancing your body's approach to aging. While cosmetic surgery may be the greatest decision for you, you need to look at the emotional side of the coin as well. There might be more to your needs than just aesthetic surgery.

Is Cosmetic Surgery a Good Choice?

There are many different sorts of cosmetic surgery that you may undergo to improve the health and beauty of your body. There is little question that you may enhance your health with a handful of these operations from an aesthetic point of view. But, before you can do so, you need to devote the time necessary to actually looking at why you want to improve. In addition, you need to discover why you wish to have this procedure in the first place.

Cosmetic surgery is necessary for some people in order to feel better about themselves. You may have a wish to only delay the indications of aging, such as those crow's feet. But, for some, the practice is done due to a lack of self-worth, which can be an issue in the long term if it is not addressed. Where do you lie? Are you looking for a few touch-ups to simply look better, or are you dealing with aging? Are you battling with your self-esteem?

There are certainly wonderful reasons to invest in cosmetic surgery. In fact, it may be a terrific way to recover some of the self-respect that has been lost. Individuals who maintain a desire to have a beautiful figure and will go to great lengths to obtain it, on the other hand, are generally insecure and, in some cases, depressed. In these circumstances, it is vital to examine why this is the case and then try to fix it.

Cosmetic surgery is a powerful anti-aging technique. But it is not the sole instrument for you. For those who do suffer from various psychological disorders, seeking support and therapy for these will allow them to feel as well as look younger. In reality, people that are well psychologically are typically able to push through health challenges and enhance their overall well-being, physically and intellectually.